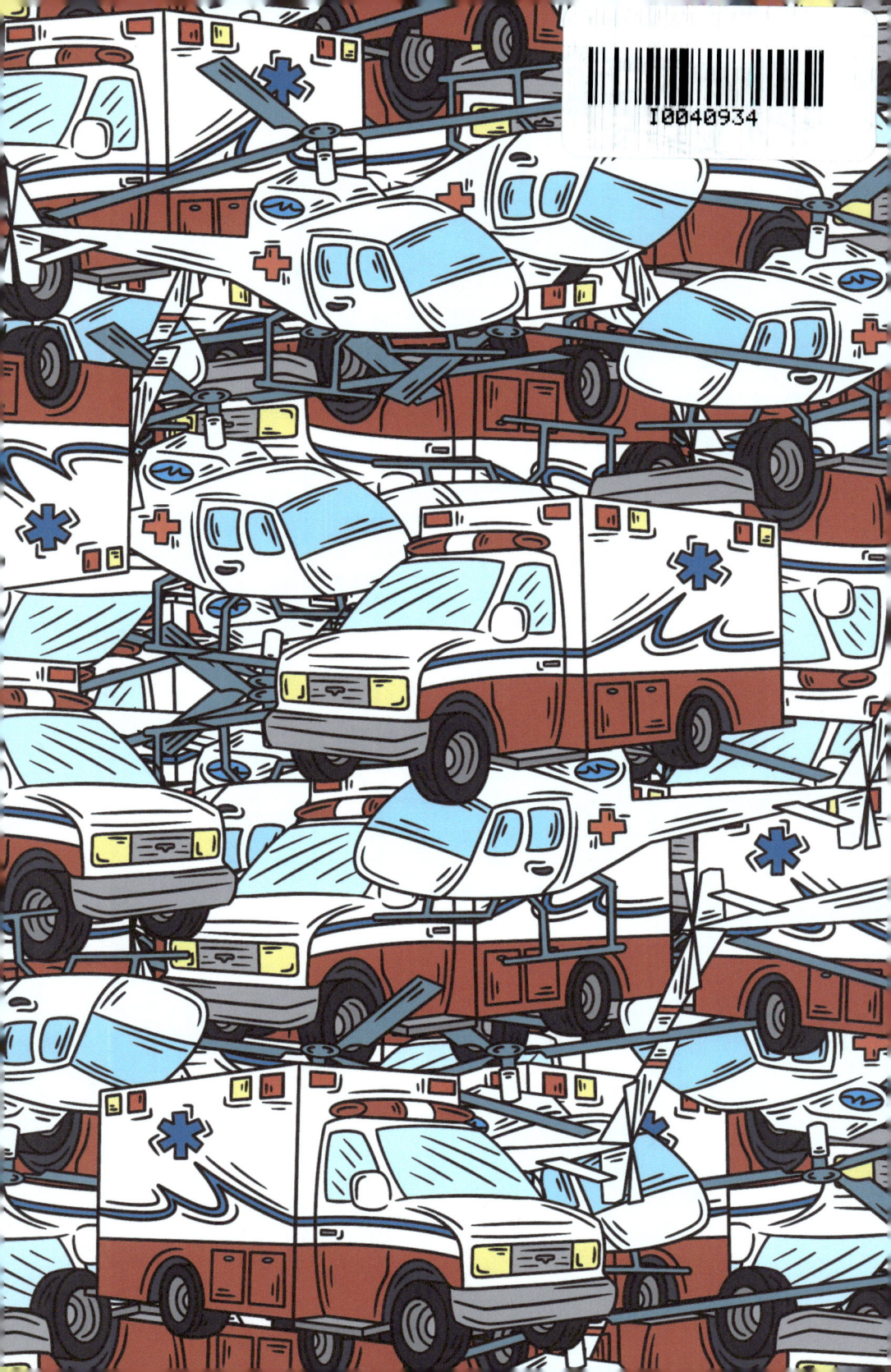

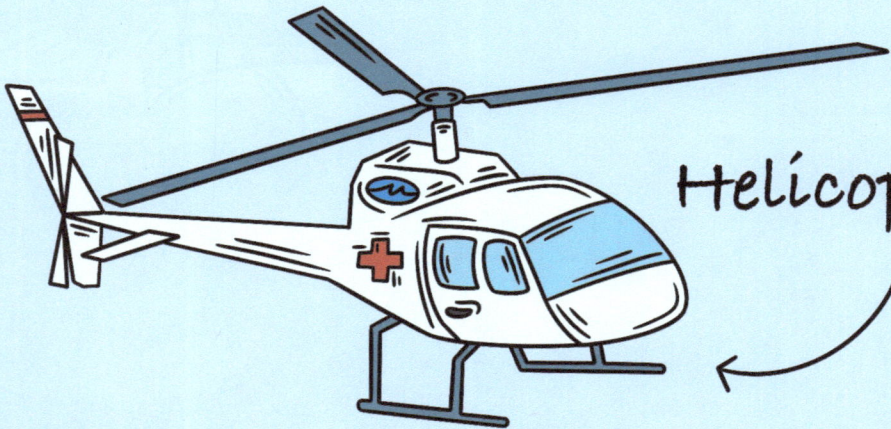

Helicopter

This book belongs to:

_____

Ambulance

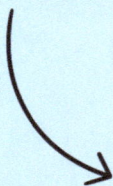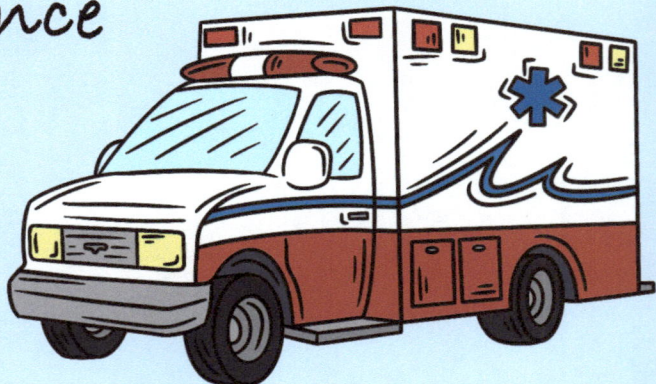

DISCOVER the STORY of

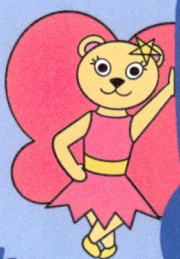

MERCY Flights

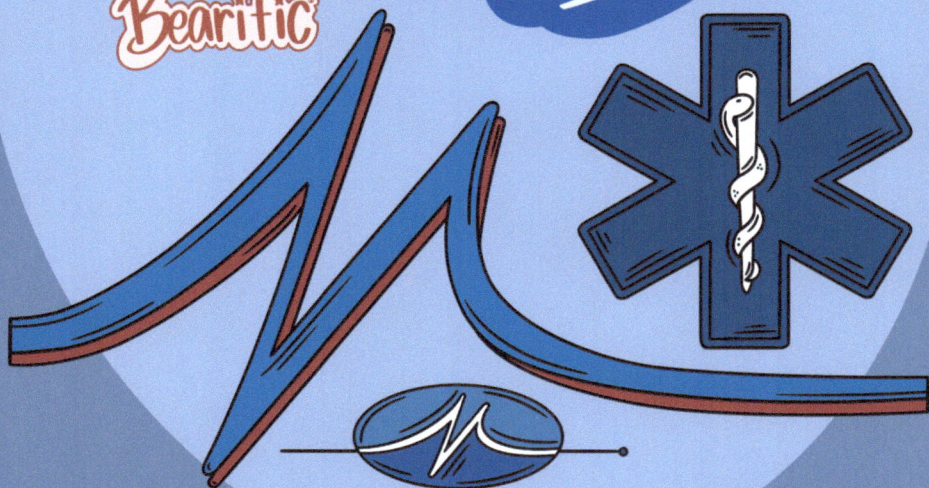

with **Bearific**®

KATELYN LONAS

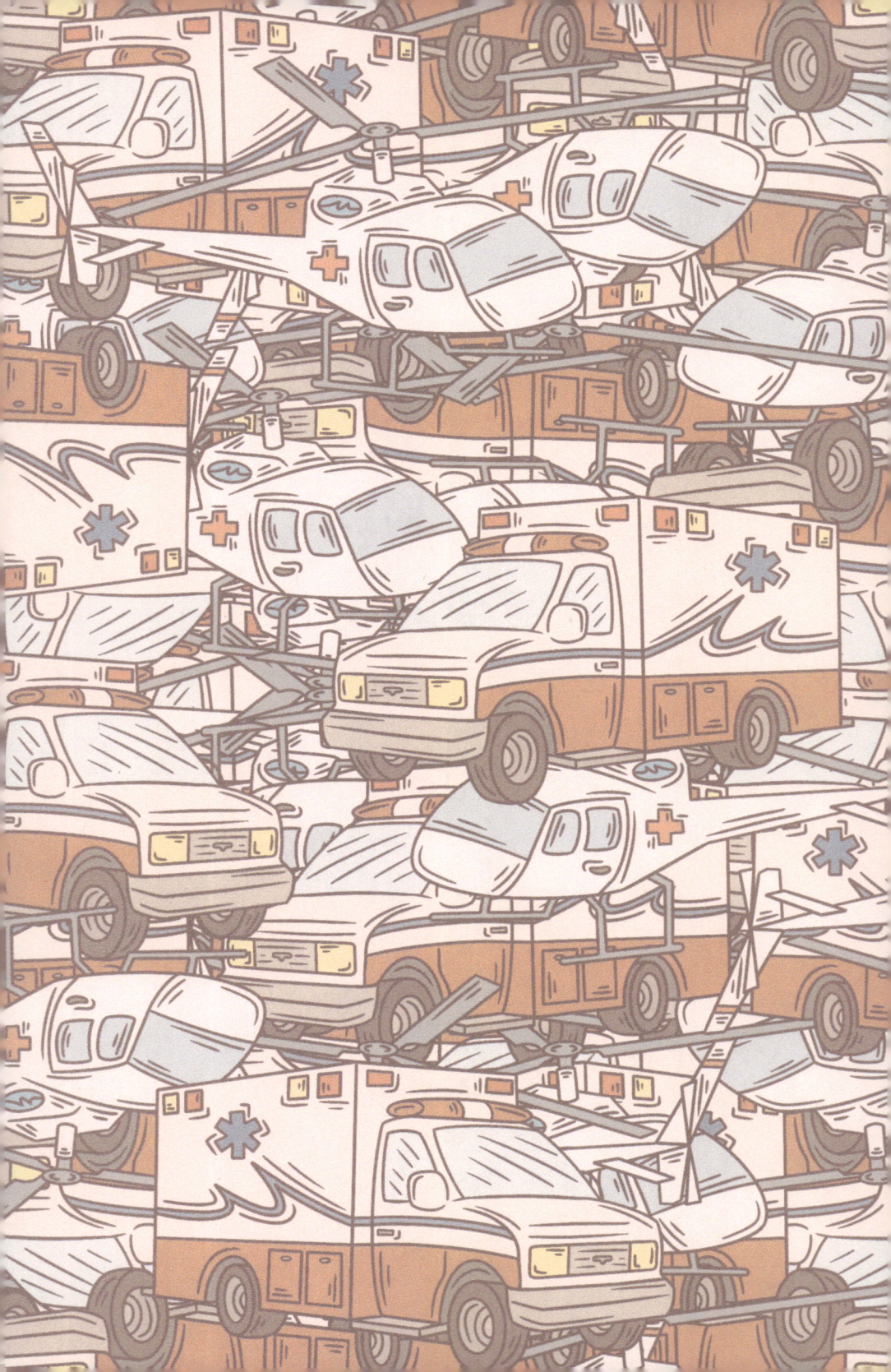

Table of Contents

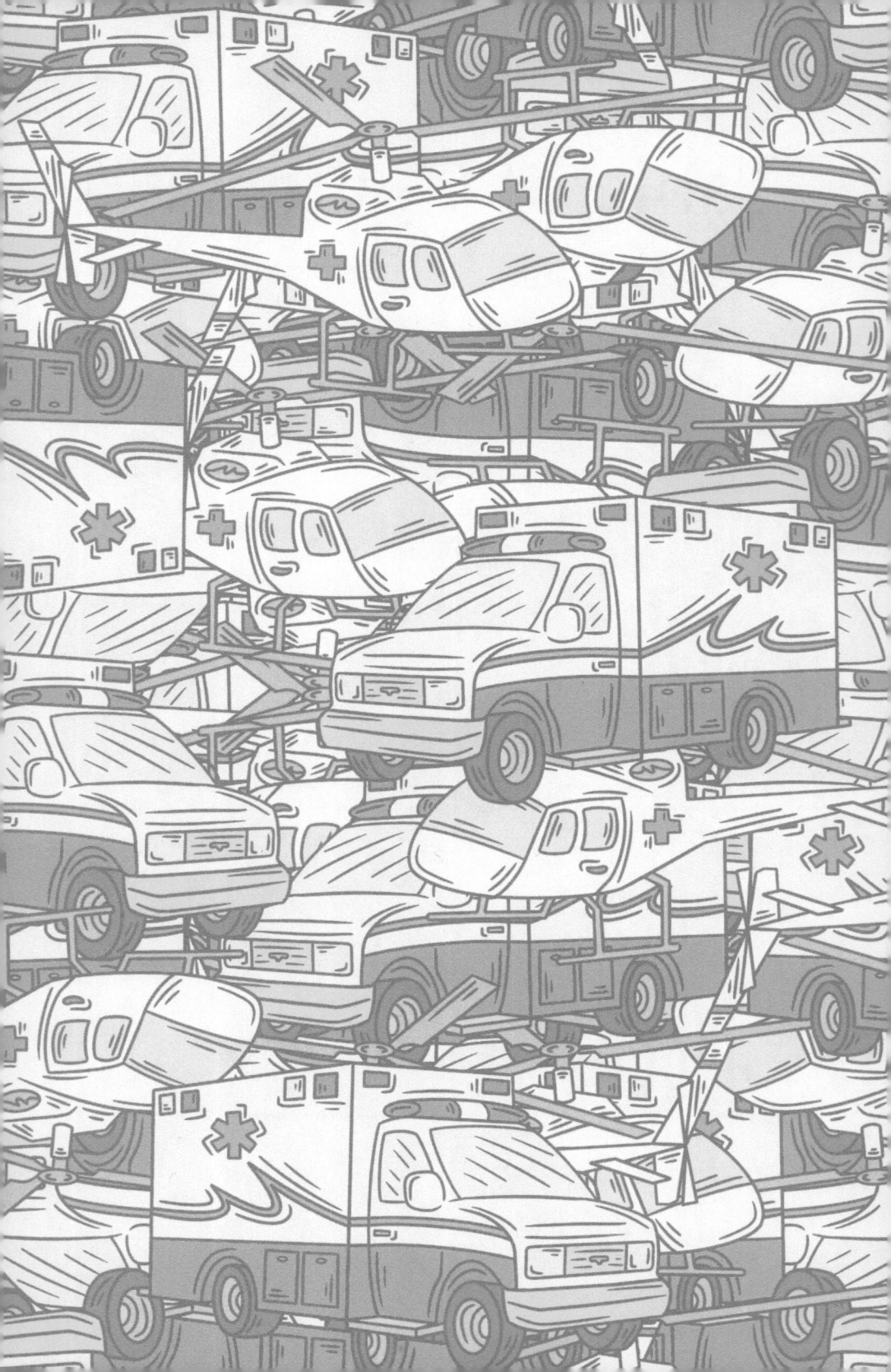

Introduction

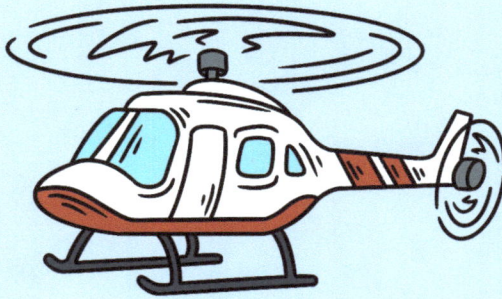

Mercy Flights is the nation's first nonprofit air ambulance service.

Since 1949, they have been striving to save lives and build healthy communities in Southern Oregon and Northern California.

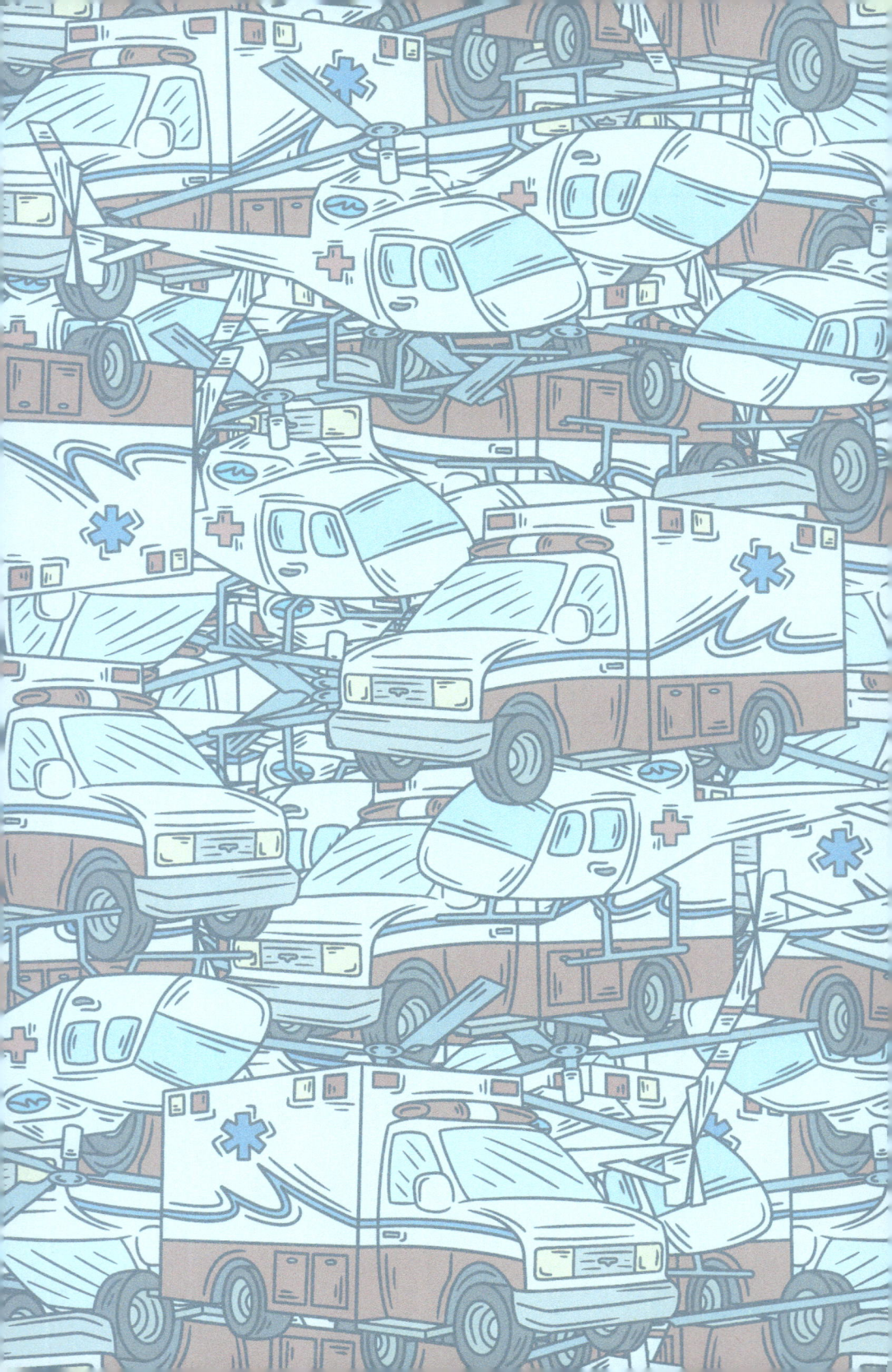

History

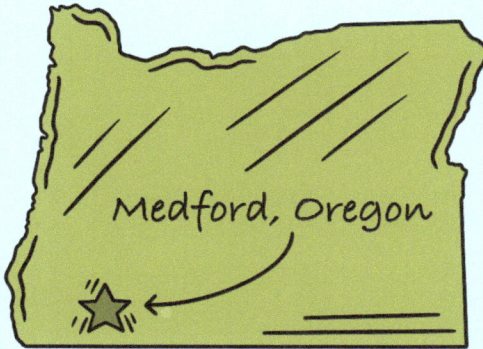

Medford, Oregon

George Milligan, an air traffic controller in Medford, Oregon, founded Mercy Flights in 1949 after a good friend of his passed away due to polio and the inability to withstand the slow ground transportation to Portland, Oregon.

Milligan raised enough money with the support of schoolchildren, scouts, and community members to purchase Mercy Flights first aircraft, a twin-engine Cessna known as the "bamboo bomber."

Twin-engine Cessna

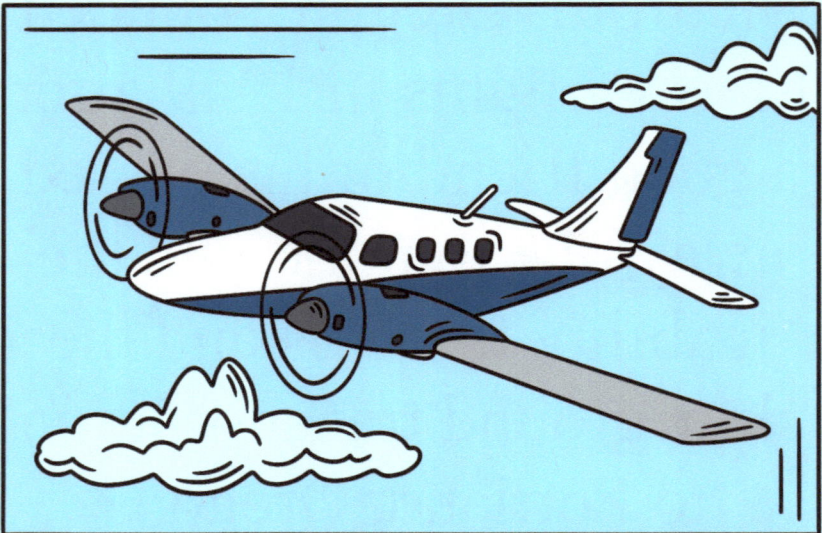

They later established a membership program that allowed community members to support Mercy Flights while guaranteeing their financial security in the event that they needed air ambulance service.

Due to increased demand, Mercy Flights added more aircraft and personnel to provide all of the medical transportation needed. As of today, they have flown over 22,000 patients.

Mercy Flights expanded its ground transportation operations in 1992 by acquiring Medford Ambulance Service and Rogue Ambulance in 1993.

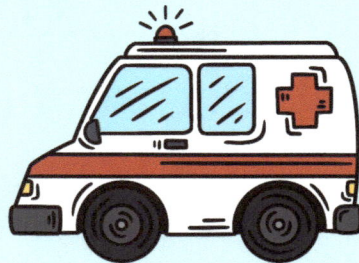

In 1995, Mercy Flights and Timberland collaborated to offer an emergency helicopter service to citizens and agencies within a 150-mile radius of Medford.

1949 August 24th: Mercy Flights was founded

Purchased First Plane "Rogue's Wings O' Mercy"

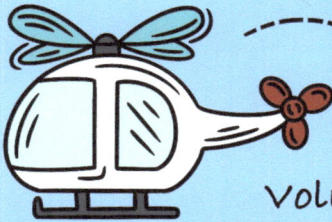

1959

Volunteers built Mercy Flights first Hangar

1992

Purchased Medford Ambulance

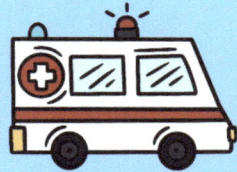

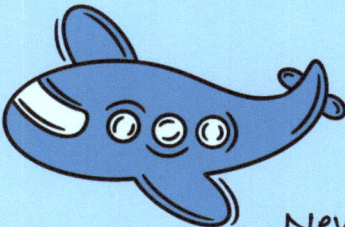

1998

New headquarters built at Medford airport

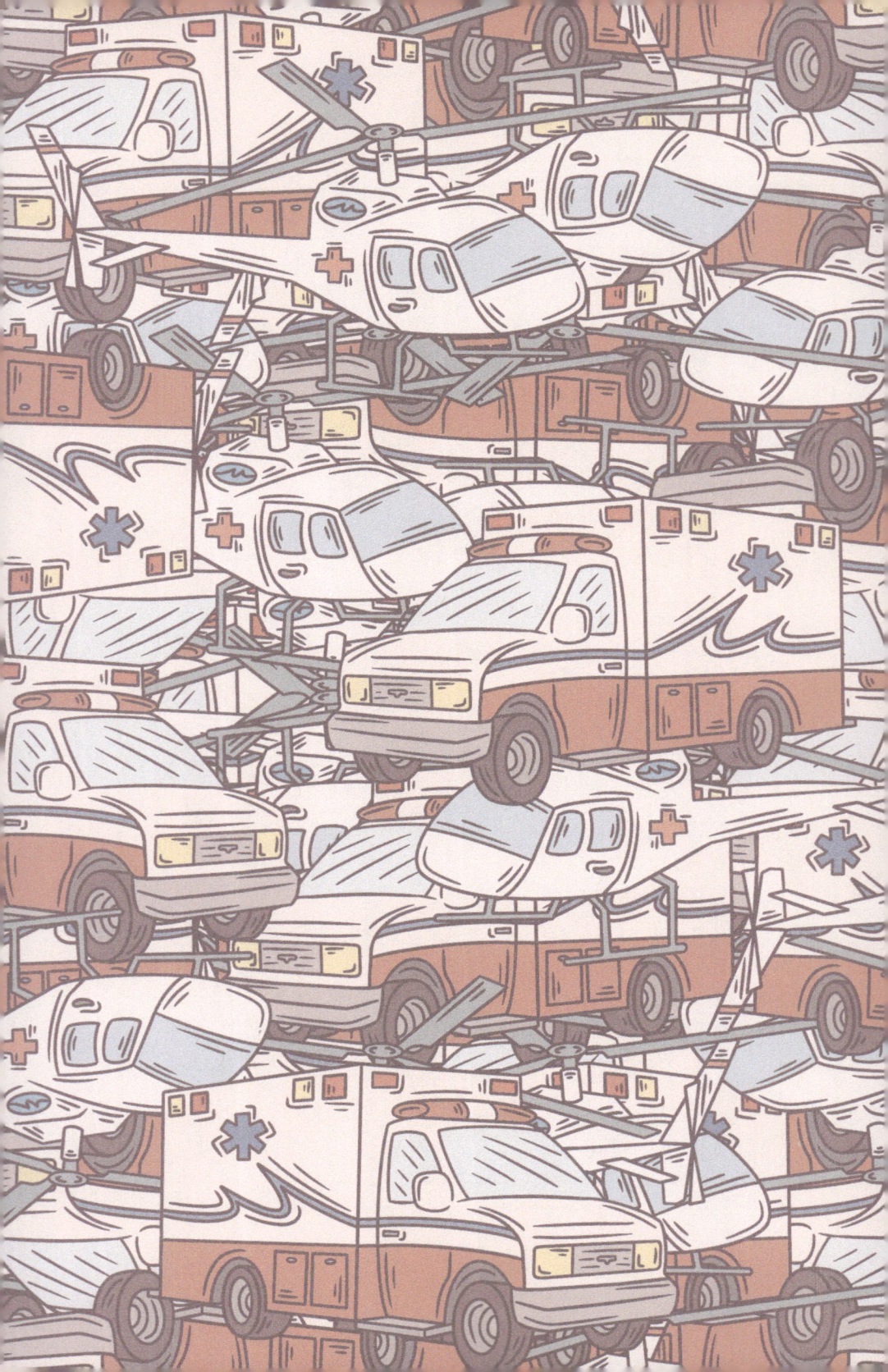

Community

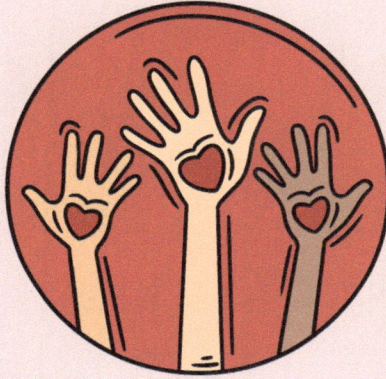

Mercy Flights is committed to providing exceptional integrated mobile prehospital care to the community.

To achieve this goal, they frequently perform safety training for community members as well as continue medical education for first response partners.

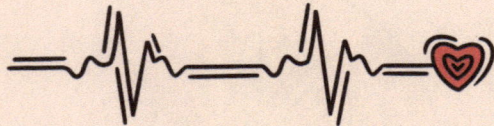

Mercy Flights operates an American Heart Association Training Site, offering training in advanced cardiac life support, basic life support, and pediatric advanced life support. Additionally, Mercy Flights collaborates with the Area Trauma Advisory Board to provide Stop the Bleed training.

Mercy Flights helps the community by providing ongoing CPR and first aid classes for a variety of programs and organizations.

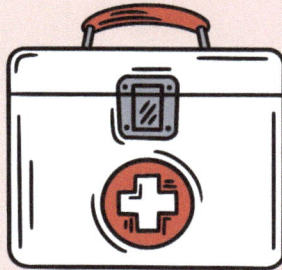

These classes are facilitated by the Mercy Flights staff and Explorer Post 131 program, which provides experience to high school students interested in professions in health care.

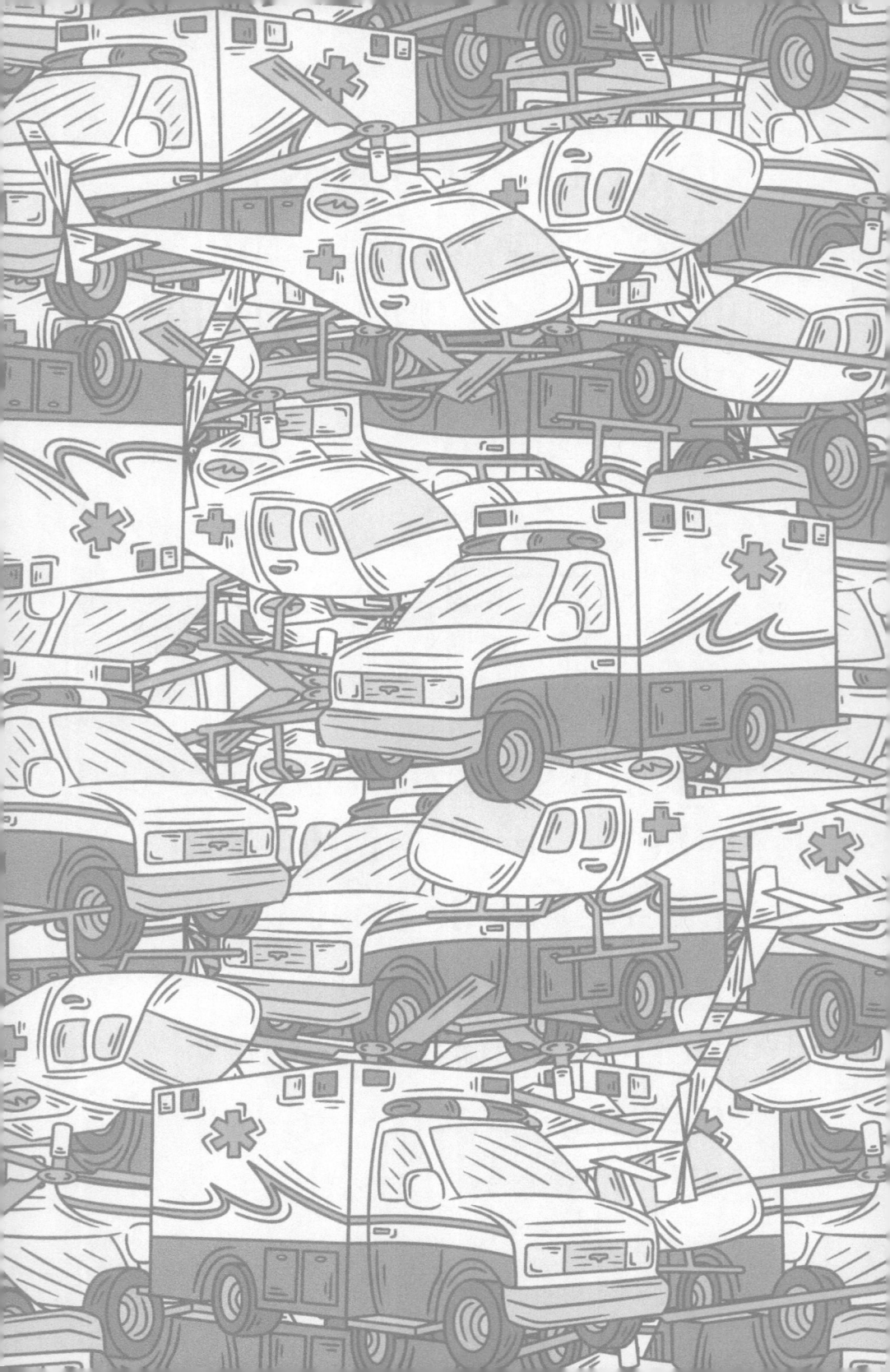

Service

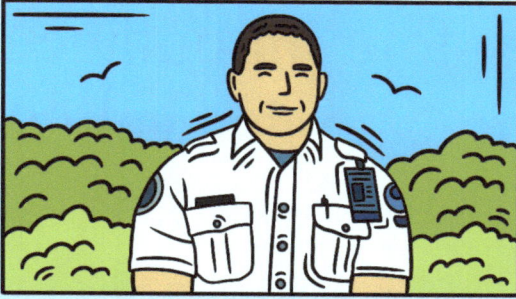

Paramedic Supervisor, Steve Lonas

Mercy Flights was started for a cause, not a profit.

Mercy Flights' dedicated healthcare professionals not only provide top-notch care for the community, they provide healthcare with compassion and heart.

As of today, Mercy Flights ground fleet consists of twenty-four ambulances and seven support vehicles.

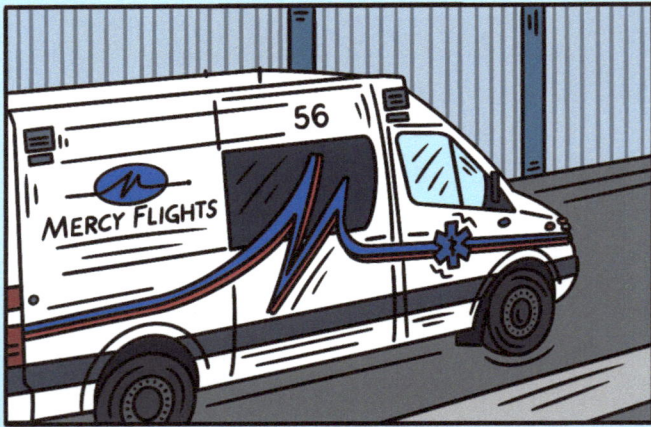

They provide ground ambulance services in over 2,000 square miles of Jackson County to anyone needing medical transportation.

Mercy Flights ground coverage area map.

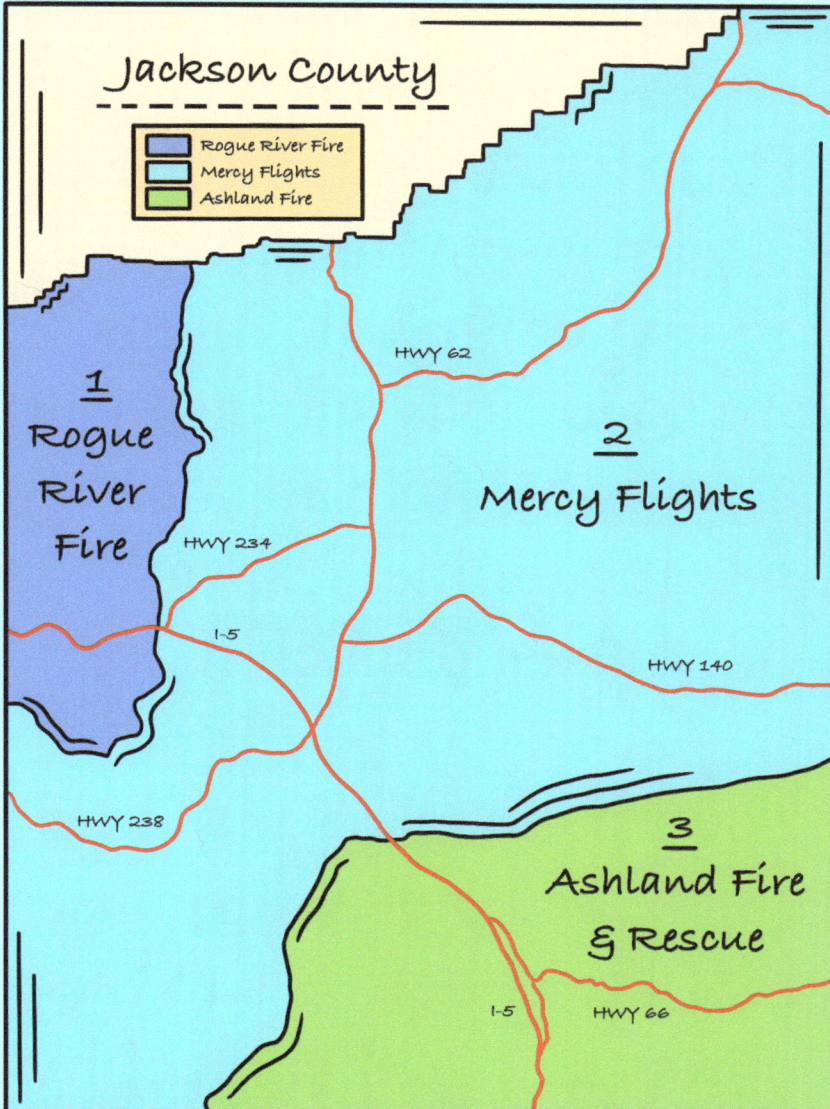

Jackson County

- Rogue River Fire
- Mercy Flights
- Ashland Fire

1
Rogue River Fire

HWY 62

2
Mercy Flights

HWY 234

I-5

HWY 140

HWY 238

3
Ashland Fire & Rescue

I-5   HWY 66

Mercy Flights offers air transport within 1,000 air miles of Medford, Oregon.

Their fixed-wing airplanes are twin-engine aircrafts equipped to handle intensive care conditions such as heart attacks, vehicle accidents, critical illnesses, sick infants, and much more.

Their helicopters provides quick emergency response and direct delivery to the appropriate medical facility.

Mercy Flights Service

Beechcraft King Air C90GTx

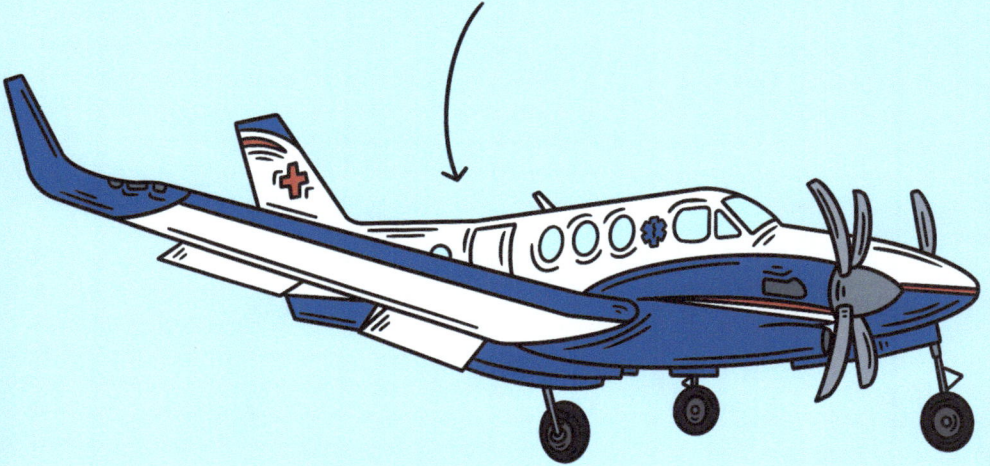

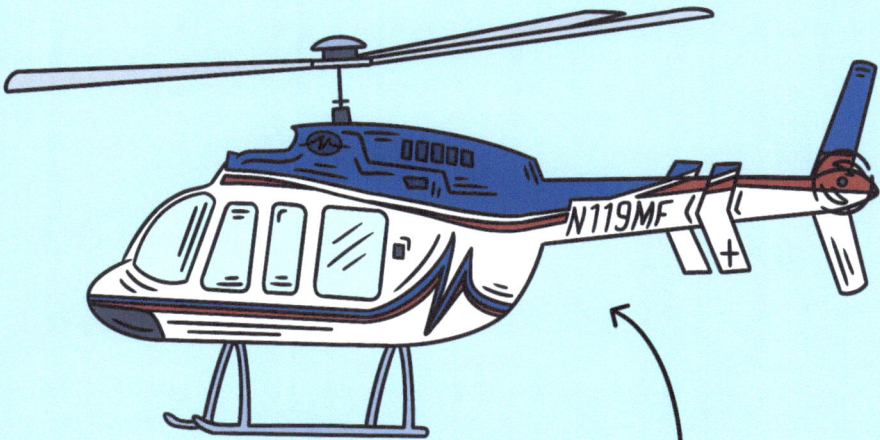

N119MF

Bell 407GX

In January 2016, Mercy Flights started the Mobile Integrated Healthcare Program.

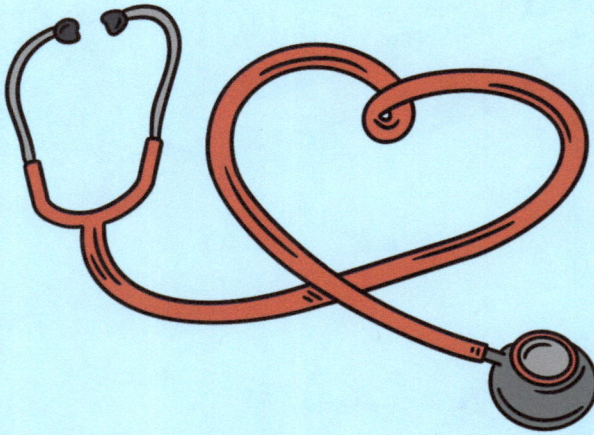

This program emphasizes the importance of improving the patient experience of care, improving the health of the population, and reducing healthcare costs.

15

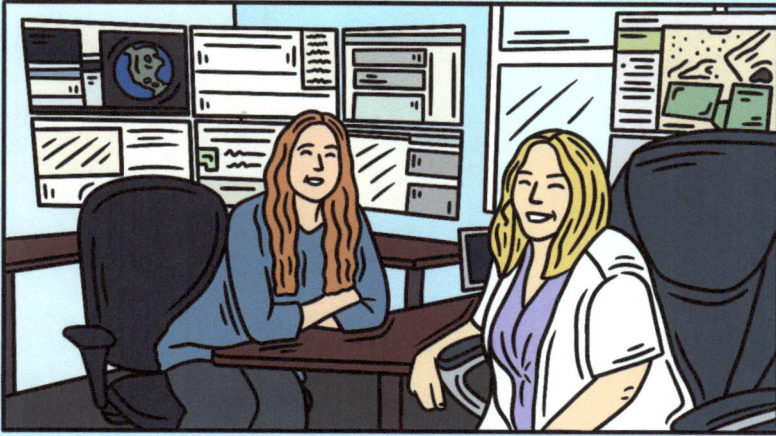

Communication Team

The Communication Center is staffed by multiple trained dispatchers who handle air and ground transportation calls as well as monitor flights.

In 2023, they managed over 32,900 calls.

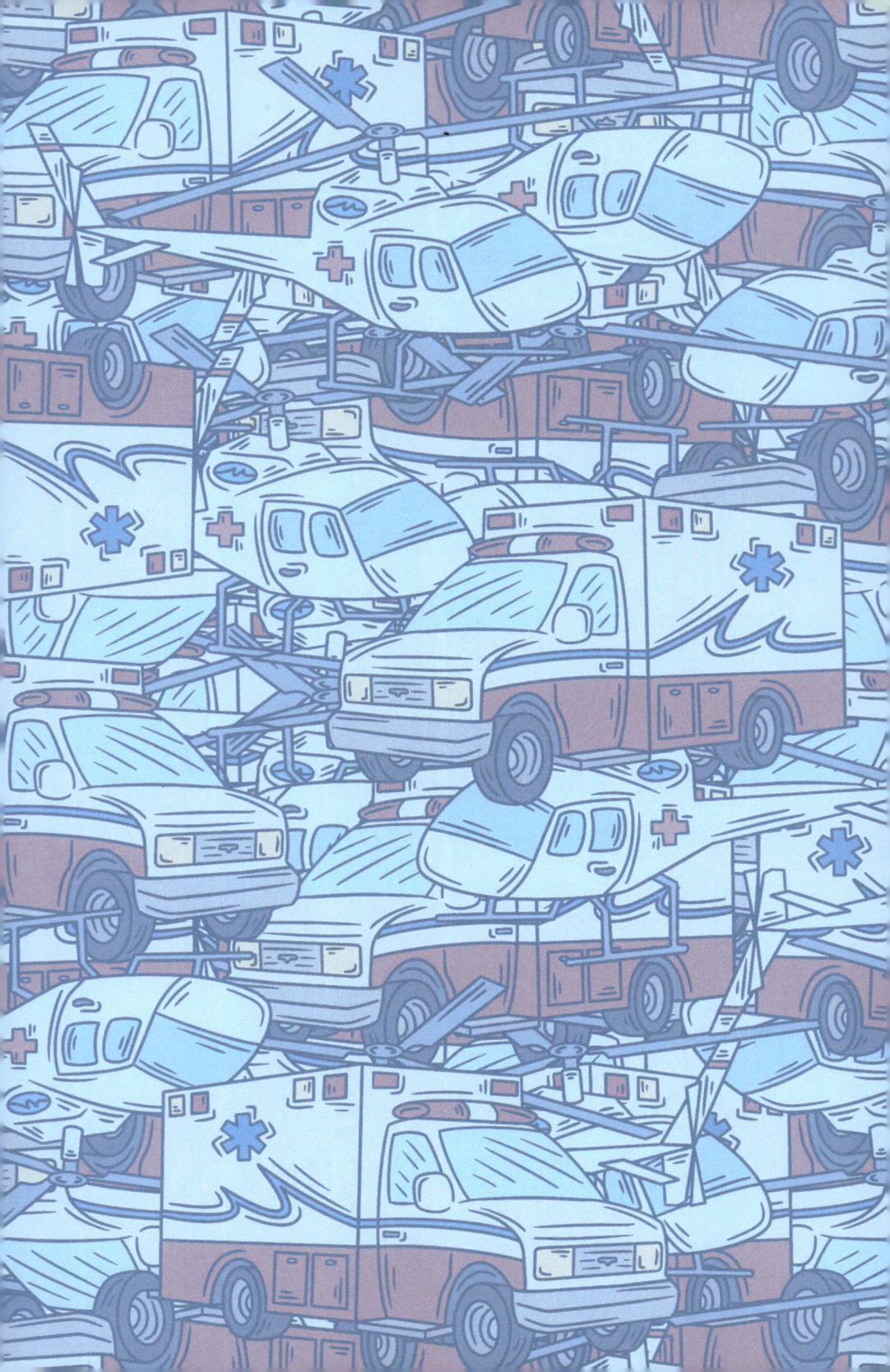

News

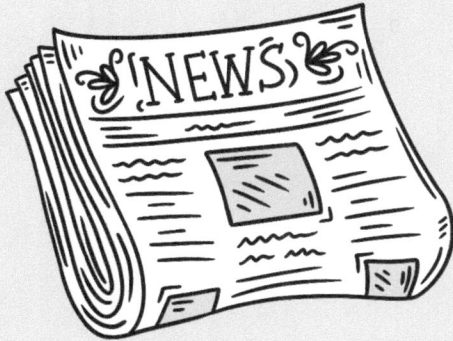

Mercy Flights was the first medical transportation organization in Southern Oregon and Northern California to carry blood on emergency aircraft and ground-based critical care ambulances. By carrying blood onboard, it increases patient survivability and provides them with a greater chance of stabilization before they arrive at the hospital.

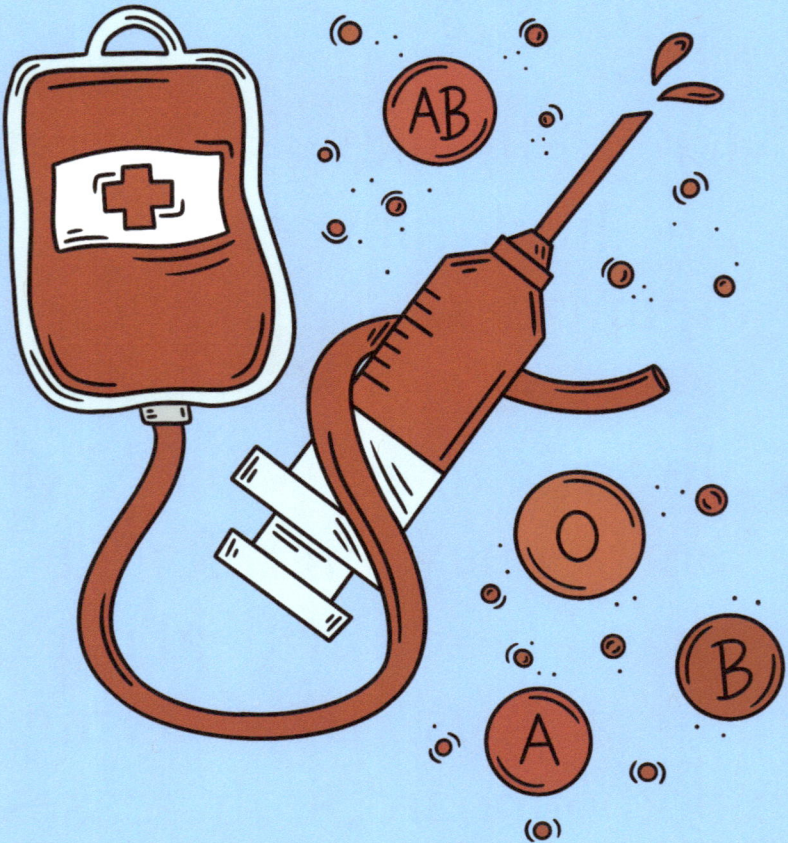

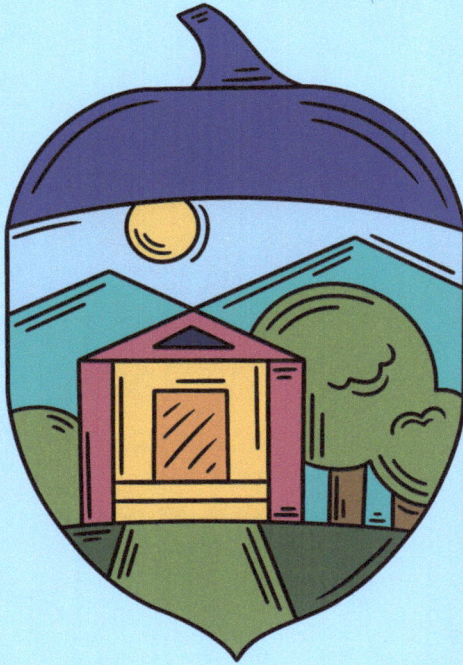

Mercy Flights also partnered with the Children's Museum of Southern Oregon to inspire children to learn and encourage interactive education with a specific focus on healthcare services.

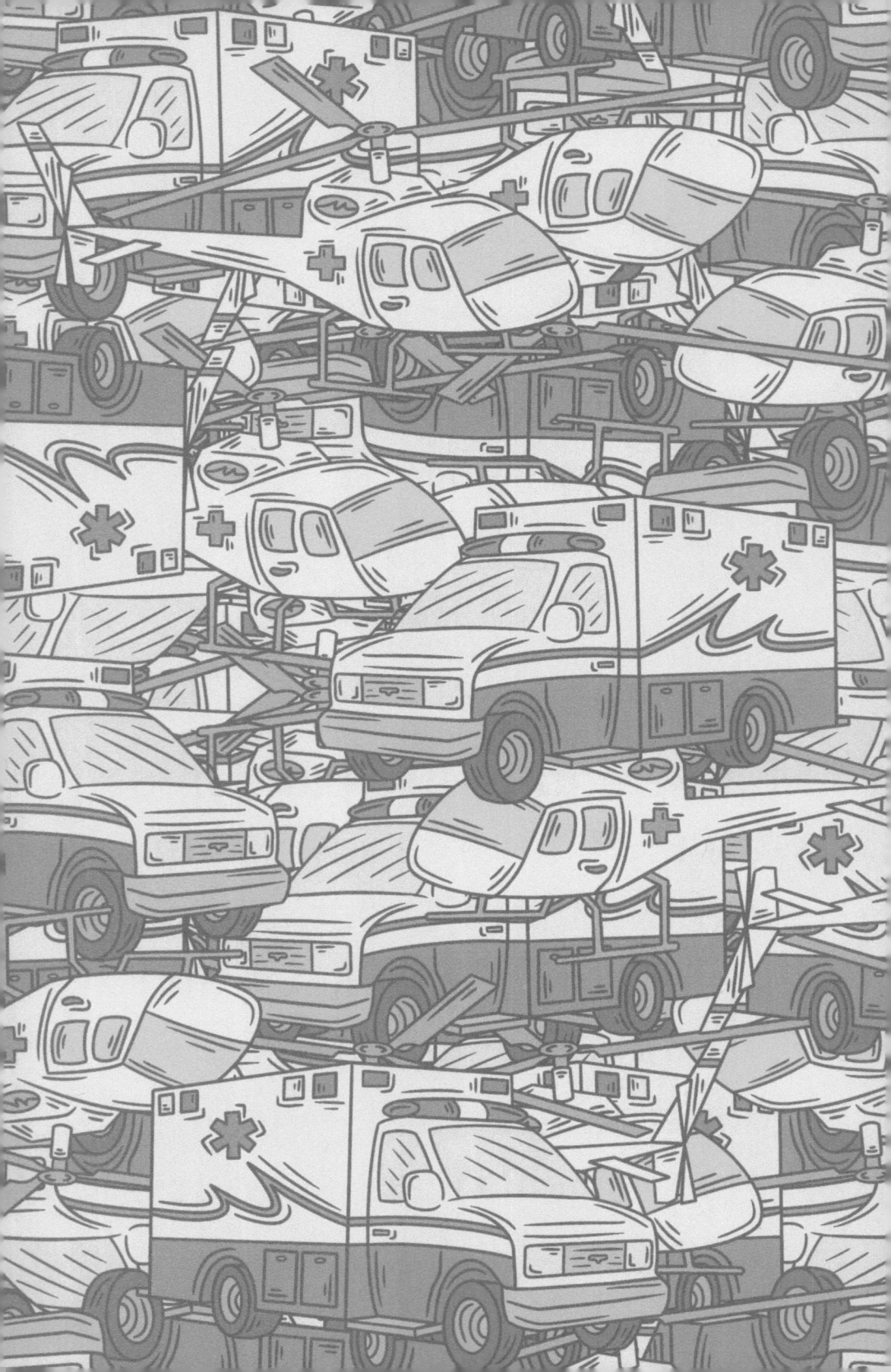

Stories

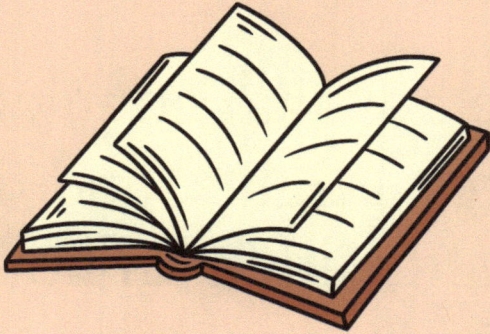

Benjamin, a 7-year-old boy, went into kidney failure due to a toxic strain of E.coli.

Unfortunately, Ben was unable to receive the necessary care in the Rogue Valley, and he required immediate transportation to

Doernbecher Children's Hospital in Portland.

The hospital contacted Mercy Flights, and they arrived within an hour to transfer Ben using a ground ambulance to the airport, where the air team would then bring him to Portland.

His family said, "We believe with all of our hearts that Mercy Flights is one of the reasons that Benjamin is still alive and thriving today."

Natalie suffered a shunt failure and was transported to Portland on multiple occasions by the Mercy Flights team.

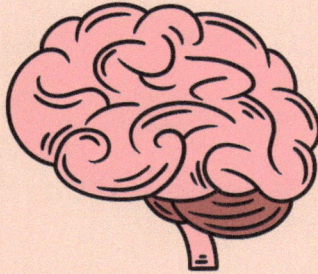

Natalie's mom said, "The Mercy Flights team was friendly and professional; they took the time to explain to a scared little girl what was going on and truly put her at ease."

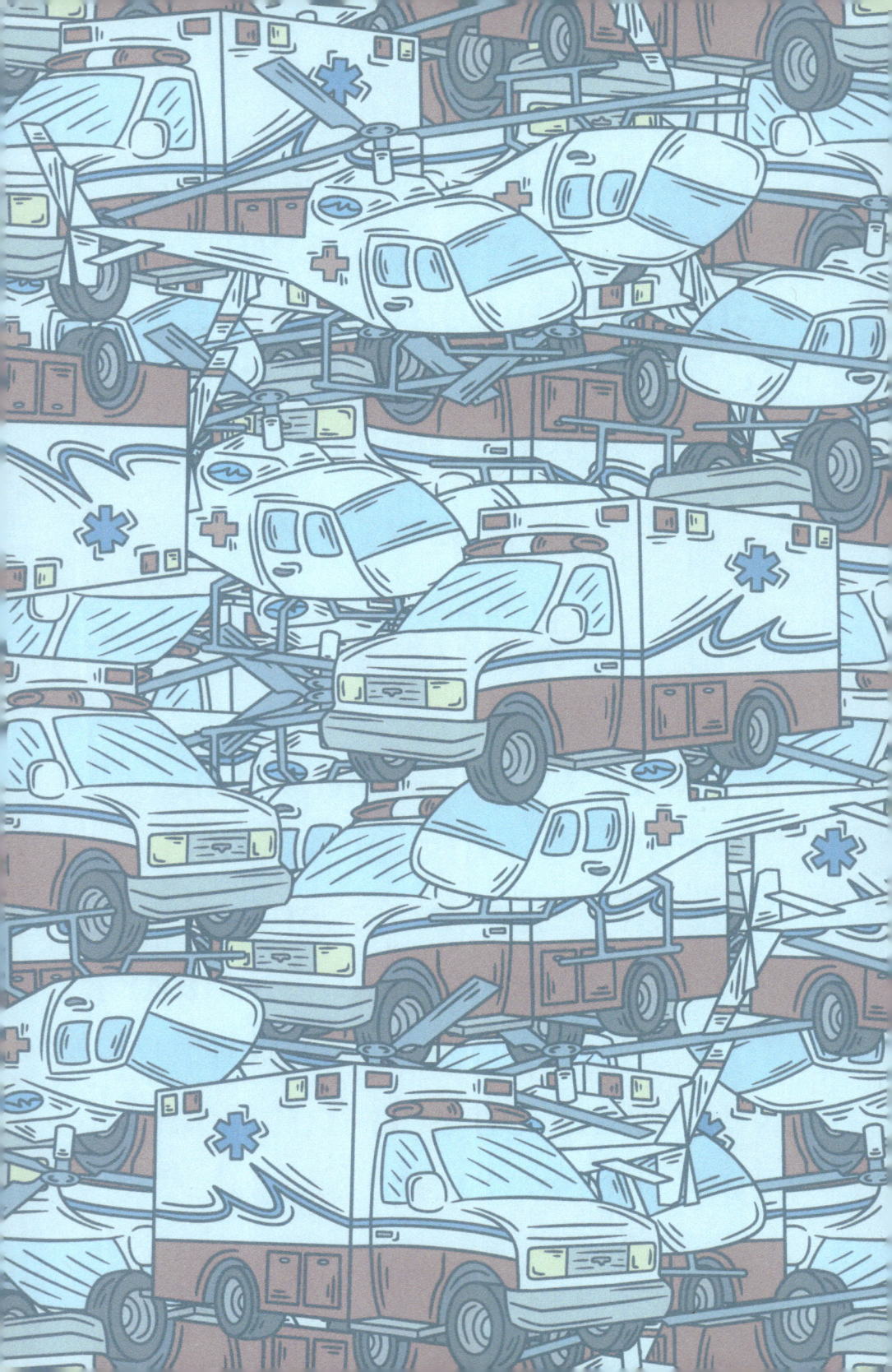

Leadership

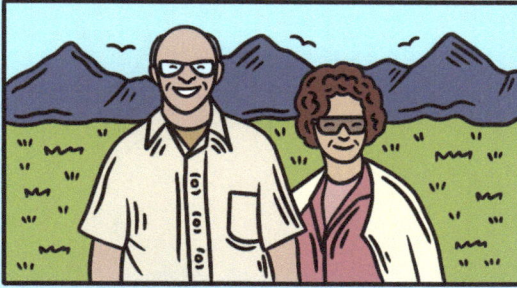

George & Helene Milligan

George Milligan sadly passed away in 1985, while his wife Helene Milligan passed away in 2019.

Mercy Flights honors them for their contributions and the positive impacts they made in the community.

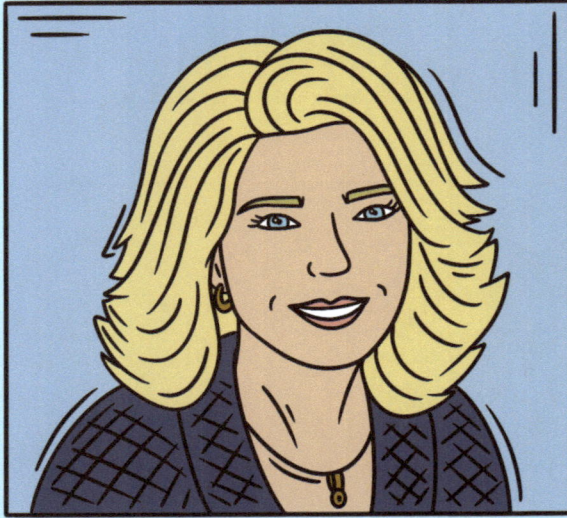

Sheila Clough is the CEO of Mercy Flights and she joined in 2020, bringing more than 28 years of healthcare leadership experience. Sheila oversees operations and administration, leading the organization's strategic planning process.

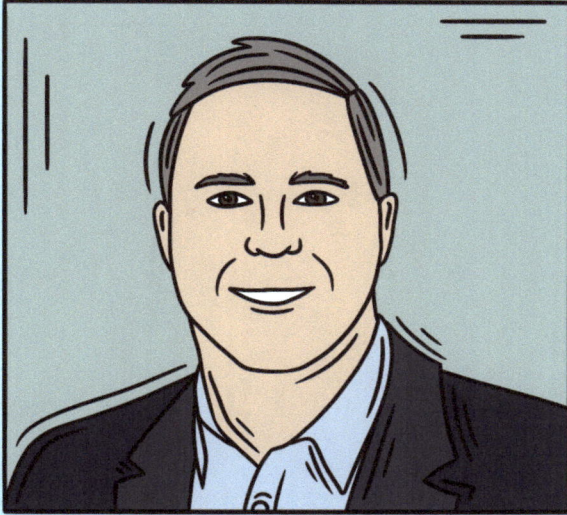

Richard Whipple is the VPO of Mercy Flights and brings over 37 years of experience in medical transportation operations. He oversees ground and flight operations and supports the strategic goals designed to improve care and service to residents.

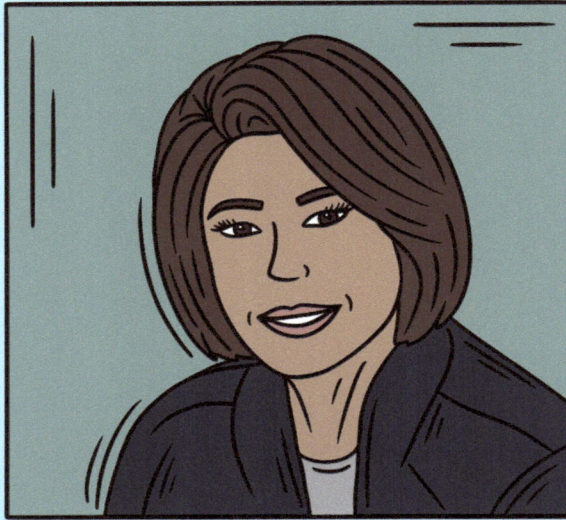

Jill Borovansky is the CFO of Mercy Flights and brings over 22 years of financial experience. She manages fiscal operations, which include billing services, payroll, accounting, telecommunication, and facility departments.

Mercy Flights board of directors include: Alan Harper, Greg Yechout, Rick Brewster, Shane Hickman, Mike Burrill Jr., Mark DiRienzo, Dr. Ed Helman, Brian McLemore, Steve Roe, Pirkko Tera, Belle Shepard & Dr. Leona O' Keefe.

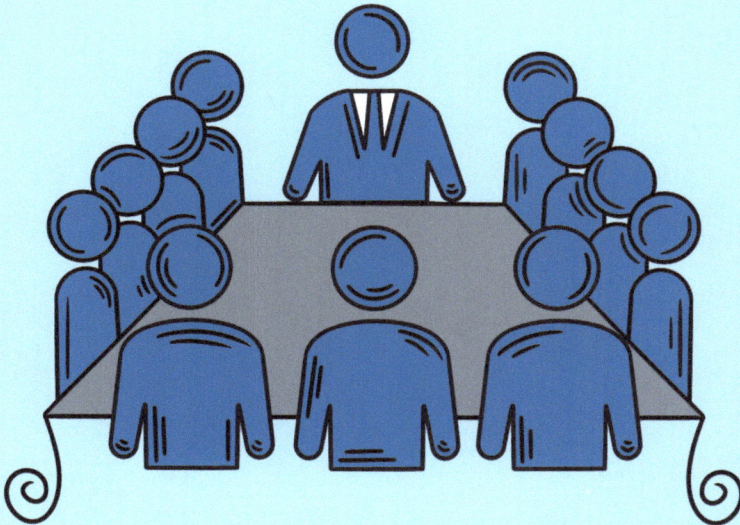

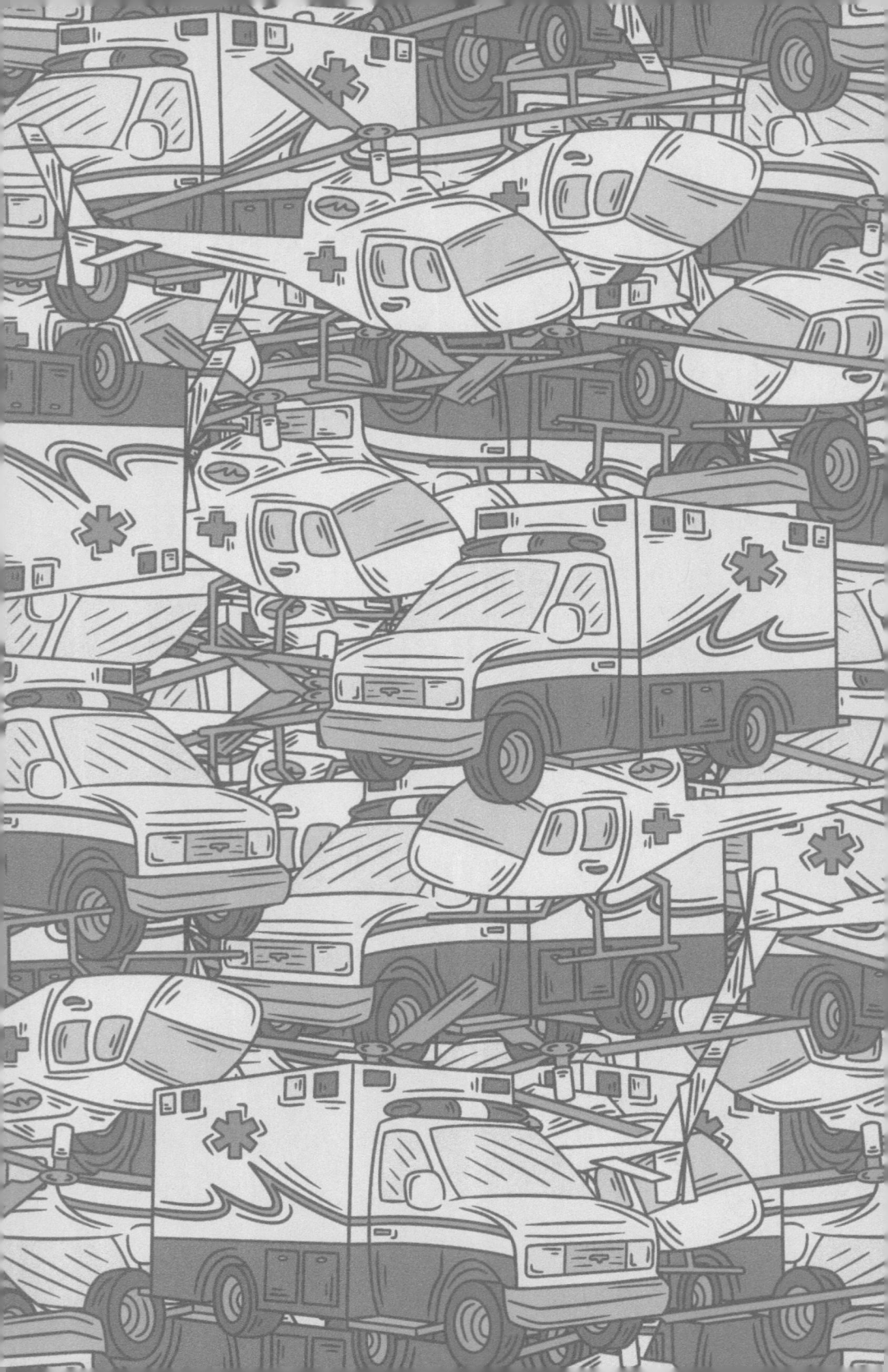

Members

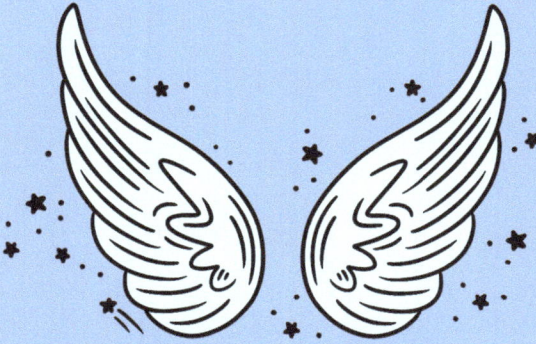

Mercy Flights has been in operation for more than 75 years and currently has over 64,000 members.

They offer air and ground lifetime memberships or yearly rates for individuals, families, groups, and seniors.

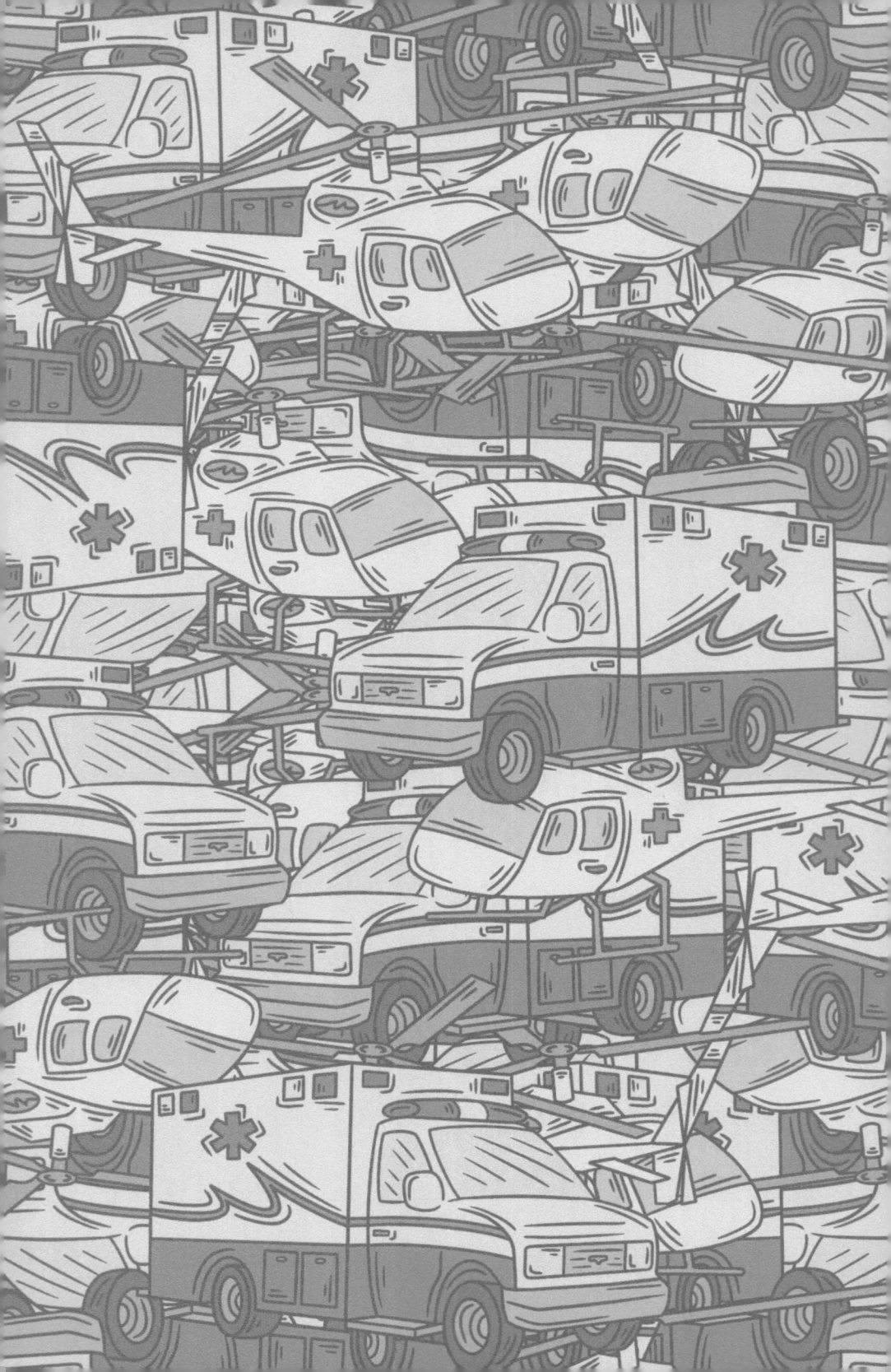

Save Lives

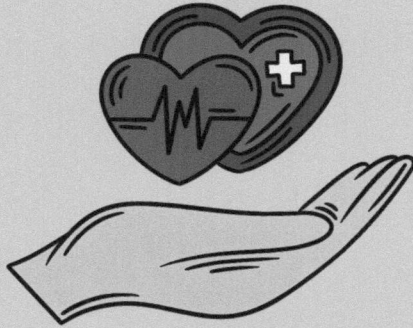

Life is precious, and having basic life-saving skills can make the greatest difference between life and death.

It's important to remember that emergencies can occur at any time, and being ready to act quickly can save lives.

Cardiopulmonary resuscitation is commonly known as CPR.

CPR maintains oxygen circulation in the body and can keep a person alive until professional help arrives.

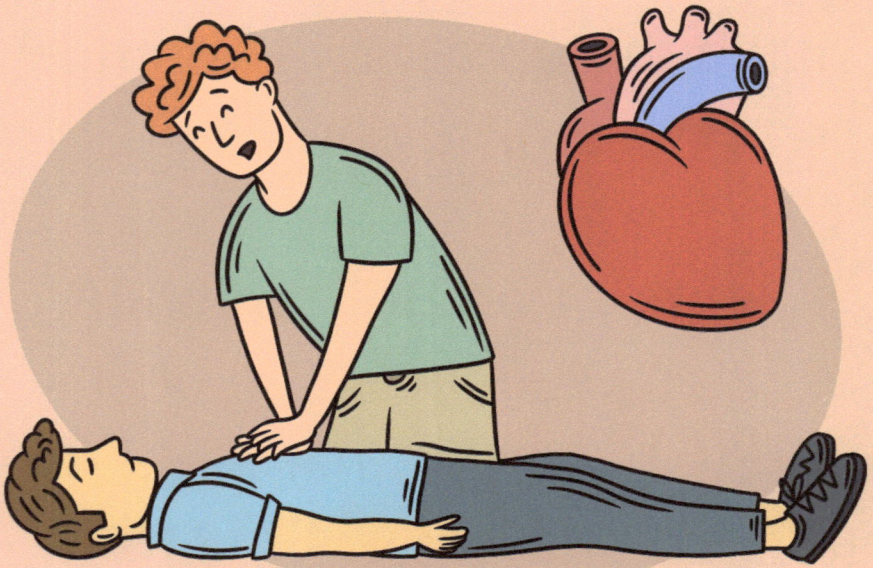

Someone may require CPR if they are unresponsive, not breathing, or have been electrocuted, near drowning, in a car accident, had a sudden cardiac arrest, or had a sudden collapse.

To perform hands-only CPR, press on the person's chest at least two inches down, at the rate of two compressions per second. Continue this until their normal heart rate restores, or emergency assistance can take over.

The Heimlich Maneuver is a technique used to help a person who is choking and cannot breathe due to a blockage in their airway caused by an object, usually food stuck in their throat.

To perform this maneuver, stand behind the choking person, wrap your arms around their waist, make a fist above their navel, grip it, and give quick, upward thrusts until the object or blockage is cleared.

The recovery position is a first aid technique used to stabilize an unconscious person, maintain an open airway, and prevent choking on vomit or saliva.

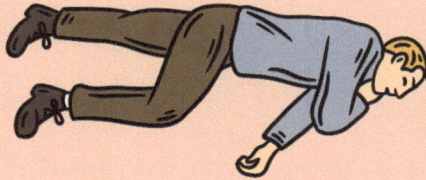

To position someone in the recovery position, lay the person on their side with their upper leg bent at a right angle. Support their head with one of their hands to keep their airway open.

If someone is experiencing severe bleeding due to an injury or wound, it's essential to take immediate action while waiting for medical help to arrive.

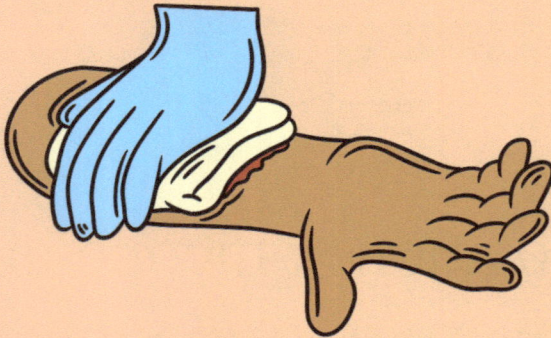

To provide first aid for severe bleeding, apply direct pressure to the bleeding wound and, if possible, elevate the injured area.

To provide first aid for a broken bone, immobilize the area by making sure that it doesn't have to support any other body parts. Then, numb the discomfort with an ice pack wrapped in a towel.

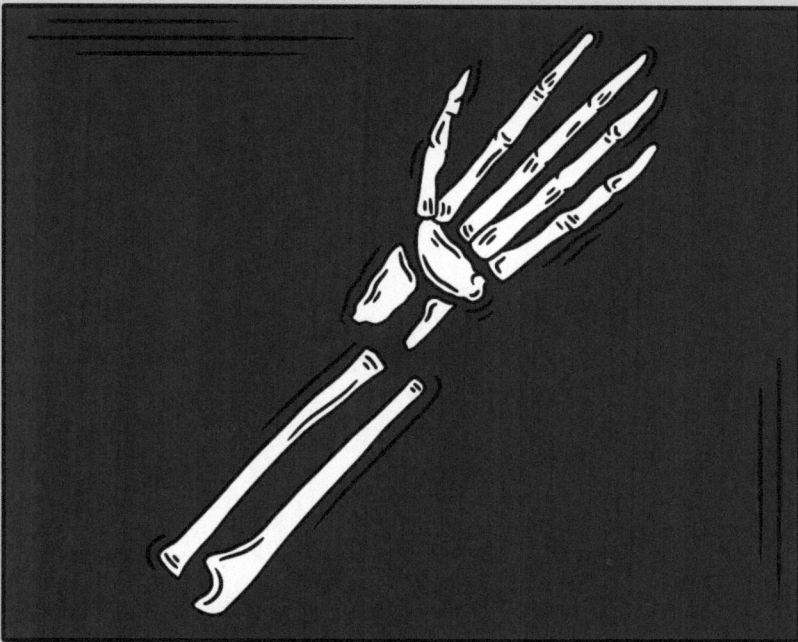

To treat first- and second-degree burns, flush the burn with cool water for at least 10 minutes. Don't use any creams or ointments on the burn. Third-degree burns should be covered with a damp cloth, and do not try to remove anything that is stuck to the burn.

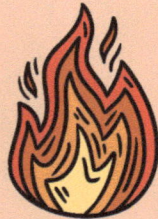

Seek medical assistance for the burn, especially third-degree burns.

The three C's of first aid are check, call, and care.

Before helping someone, check your surroundings to ensure you are not putting yourself in danger. Then call for medical assistance. You can help care for them by offering support, staying calm, and being reassuring.

If you are treating burns or bleeding wounds, wear gloves to protect yourself from blood-borne viruses.

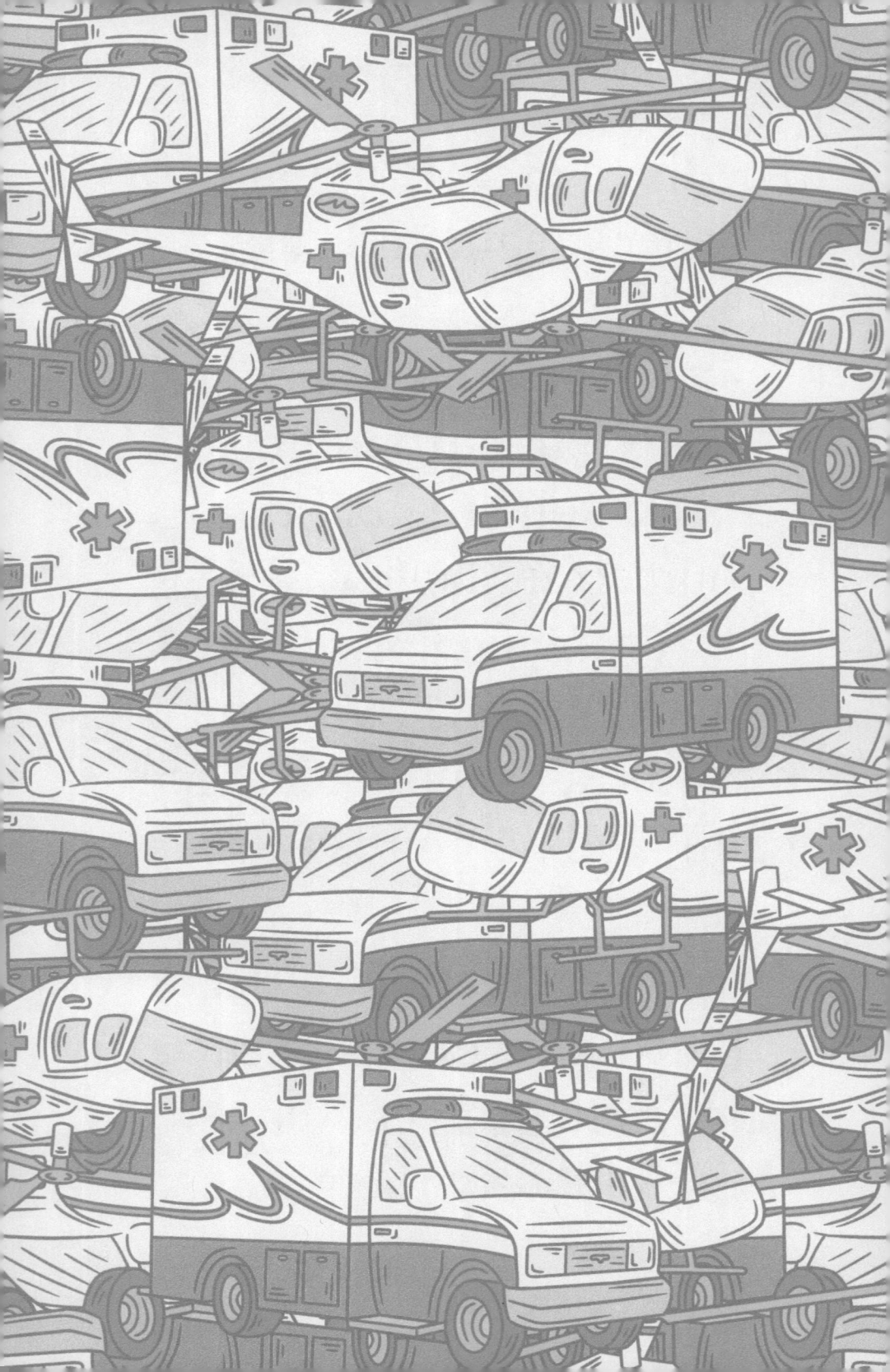

Pictures

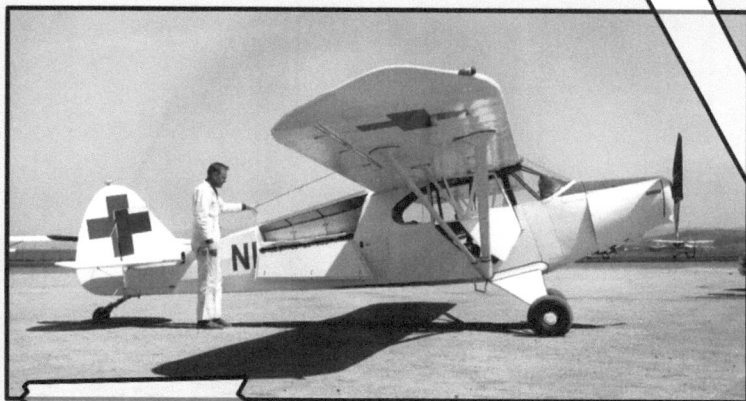

The beginning of Mercy Flights.

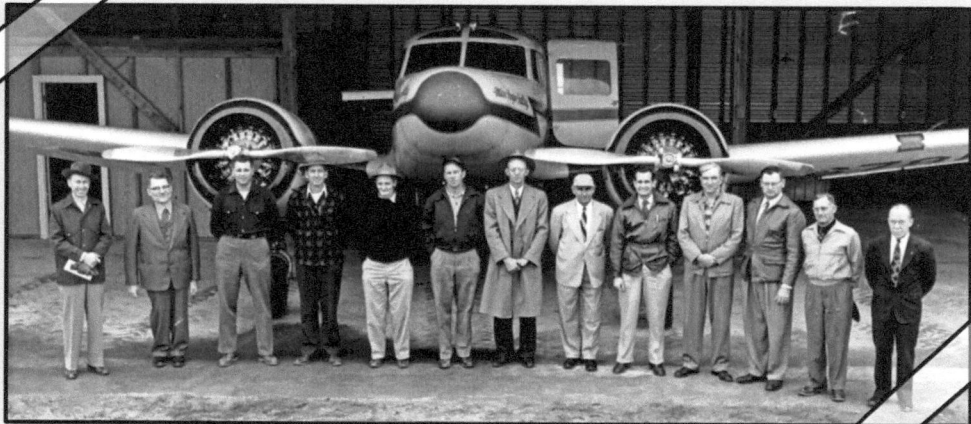

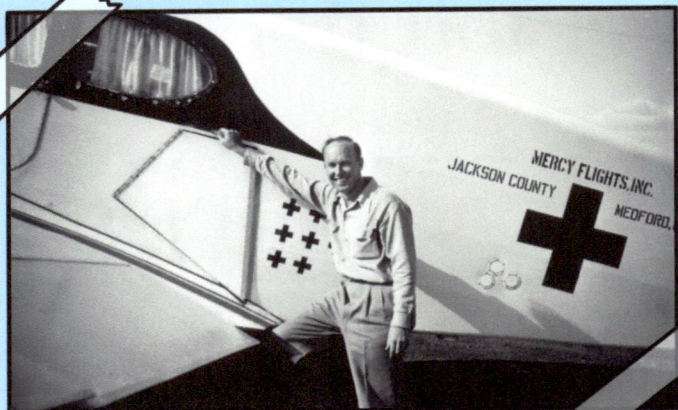

The founder George Milligan.

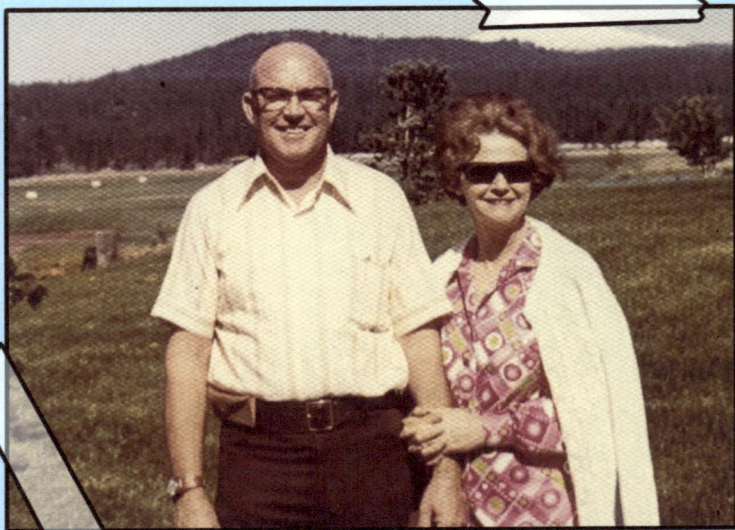

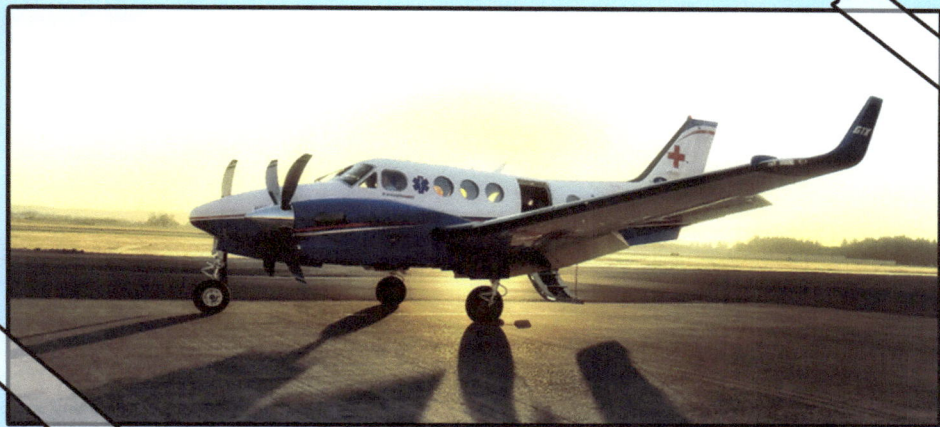

Mercy Flights plane and helicopter.

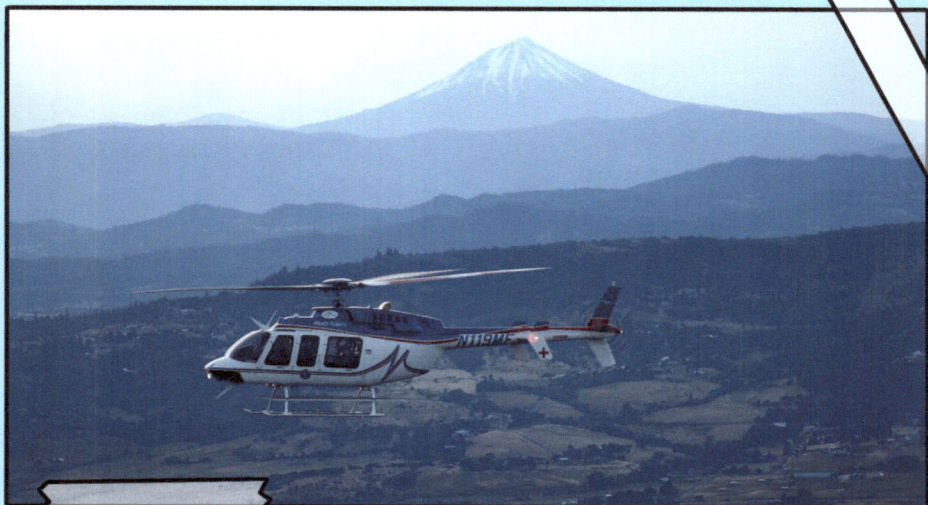

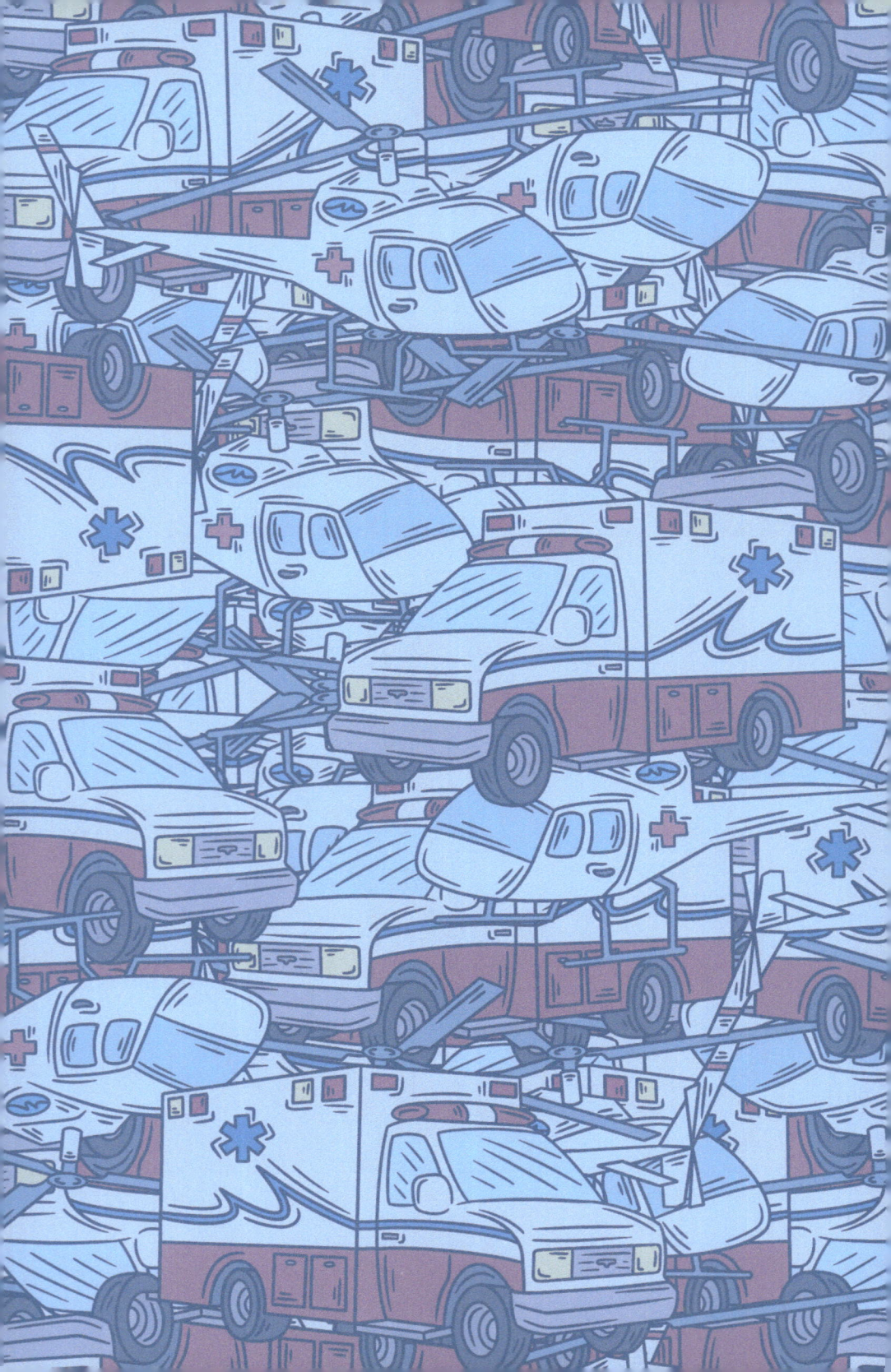

Activities

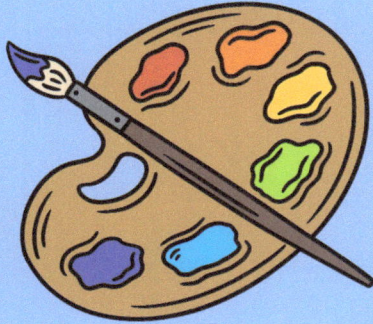

Get ready to do some fun activities such as coloring and problem solving with Mercy Flights.

Grab your crayons, markers, and colored pencils to show your creativity and let your imagination fly.

- Mercy Flights Word Search -

```
N T B A N D A G E E J K E D V
X Y J P J H E A L T H B F O D
H E L I C O P T E R O G K F O
B J F H Y M E V R F L I I N C
X I F T H E R M O M E T E R T
P E R P P N G N X C V M G S O
A P T J K Y K U T T G H B A R
R M E R C Y F L I G H T S F Z
A V R A U G A I R P L A N E N
M I N H O S P I T A L M X T U
E R S T E T H O S C O P E Y R
D U A M B U L A N C E O L A S
I S N O T Y M C R M F A D H E
C E V Q J L M E D I C I N E G
B U V I V U Z Q Z O A H A X H
```

Mercy Flights	Stethoscope	Thermometer
Helicopter	Ambulance	Paramedic
Airplane	Hospital	Medicine
Bandage	Health	Doctor
Safety	Virus	Nurse

- Mercy Flights Coloring -

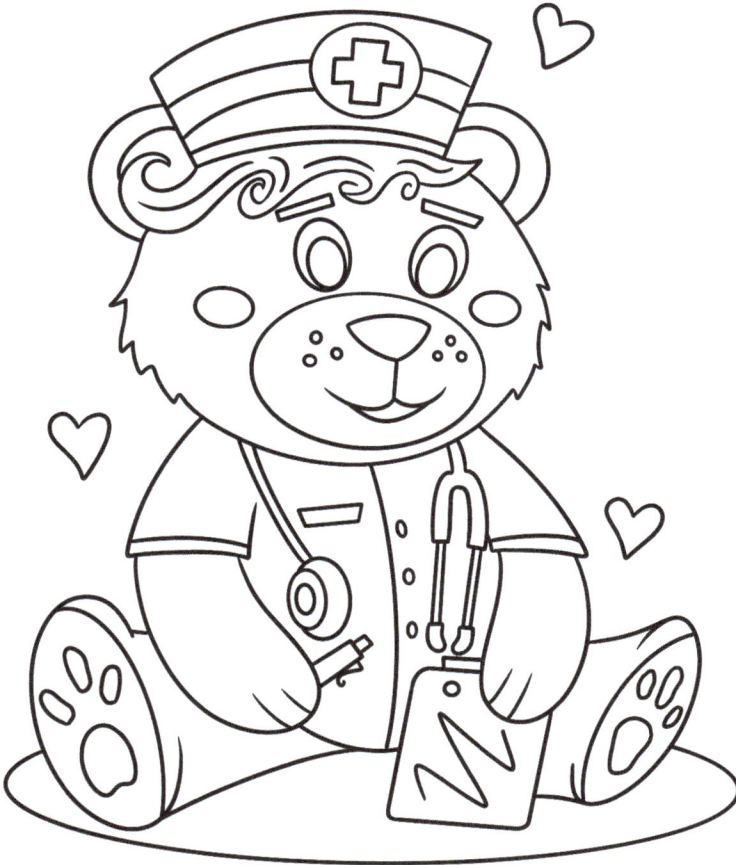

- Mercy Flights Maze -

- Mercy Flights Crossword -

Look at the image to determine the word.

ANSWER KEY

Down:

1.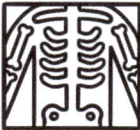

2.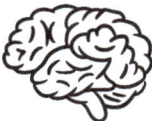

Across:

2.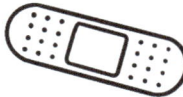

3.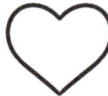

4.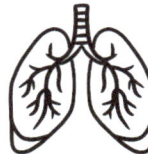

More of Mercy Flights can
be found on Instagram and
Facebook. Their website is
www.mercyflights.com

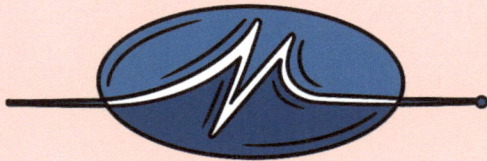

Contact Mercy Flights.
For membership, billing,
and general information, call
541-858-2600. For hospital
and medical transports, call
541-779-6551.

Address: 2020 Milligan Way
Medford, OR 97504

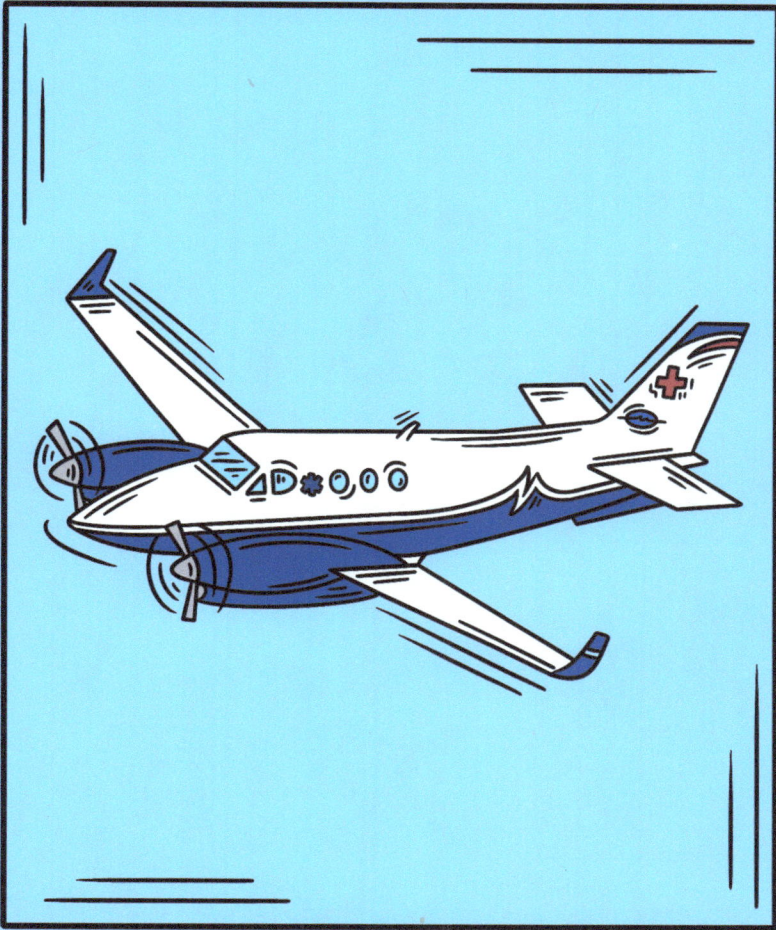

"The nation's first
nonprofit air ambulance."

- Mercy Flights -

The End!

remember to:

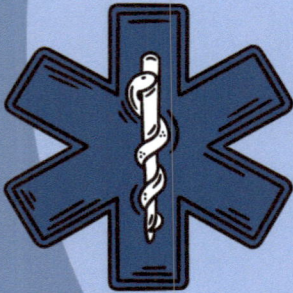

BELIEVE
DREAM
ACHIEVE

Author & Illustrator

Katelyn Lonas

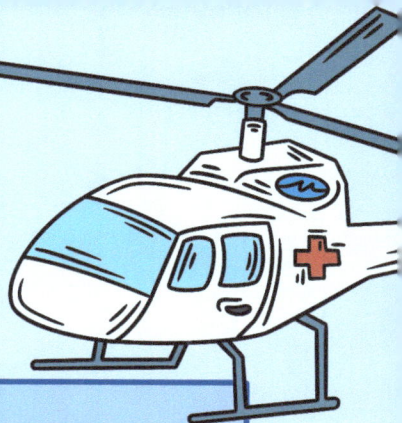

Katelyn is 17 years old and resides in Southern California. Katelyn loves to encourage others to always believe in themselves and chase after their dreams! She began writing and illustrating her first book at age 9 and went on to publish 69 more books. She hopes you enjoyed this book and are excited for more to come!

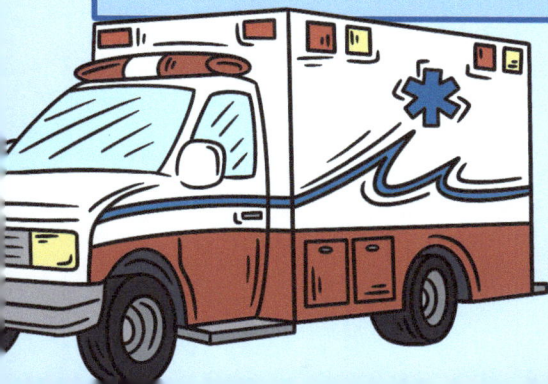

-Katelyn Lonas

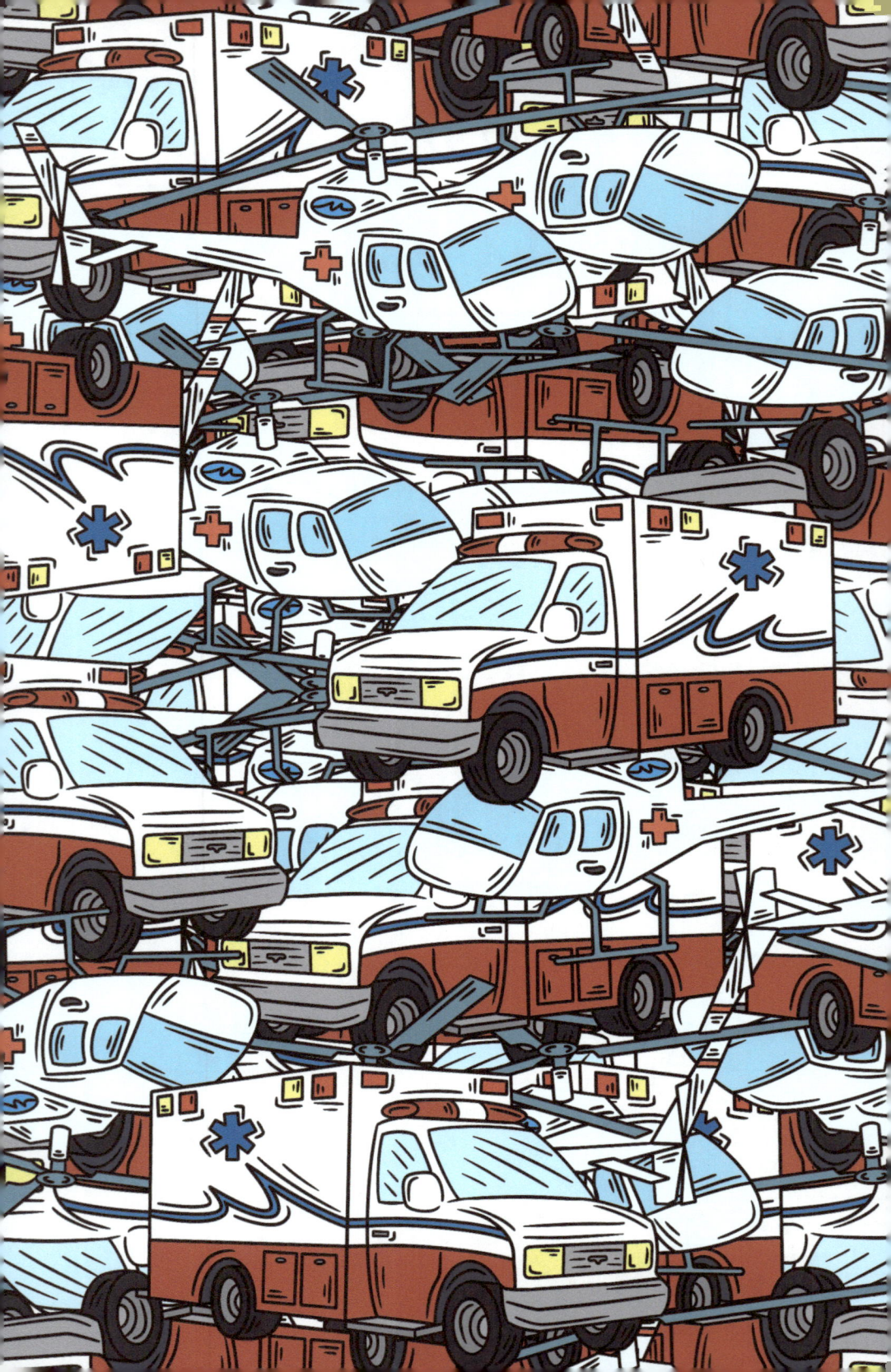

www.ingramcontent.com/pod-product-compliance
Lightning Source LLC
Chambersburg PA
CBHW041714200326
41519CB00001B/166